The Complete Clean Eating Cookbook

Ketogenic cleanse, restore metabolism with tasty whole-grain recipes and programs for healthy everyday meals

TABLE OF CONTENTS

Introduction

Healthy eating is essential for everyone. At clean eating meal prep we understand that everyone has different needs, goals, and preferences. That is why we provide healthy eating meal prep options for individuals to choose from.

Our meal prep options come in the form of ready-to-eat and store-ready meals. They include a wide variety of lean proteins and vegetables. The store-ready items can be picked up at your local grocery store, while the ready-to-eat items are made fresh and frozen daily in our facility.

We put a lot of thought into how to make our meal prep items healthy and appealing while still being easy to prepare. That is why we use no additives or preservatives in our meal prep products. We are committed to providing you with clean, delicious meals every time you order from us.

We all know that a healthy diet is key to maintaining a healthy lifestyle. clean eating meal prep knows that a healthy diet can also be great when you're on the go. That's why we created meal prep kits to help you stay on track with your clean eating goals.

With the clean eating meal prep meal prep kit, you can prepare and store everything you need for your clean eating regimen in one convenient location. You'll be ahead of the game because you'll be prepared for that busy day when you're running around after school, work, or your kids.

Preparing your meals ahead of time will eliminate the temptation to order take out and save yourself from being hungry and unfocused during the day. Plus, it will save you money as well!

"But I don't eat healthy! I need something convenient!" You're not alone.

We get it. Everyone wants to eat healthy without sacrificing the ability to make delicious, nutritious meals.

At clean eating meal prep, we understand. That's why we've created a new meal prep service that makes eating healthy easy to do.

What is Meal Prep? How Does It Work?

Meal prepping is the process of creating an entire day's worth of healthy and nutritious meals ahead of time. This way you can focus on shopping for ingredients, rather than what you plan to cook. Yes, you can still order delivery or eat out, but it is so much easier to make the whole meal at once!

Meal prepping allows you to eat healthy with a lot more flexibility! So say goodbye to go-to foods that are high in refined carbs or just generally unhealthy and hello to fresh, new options!

Being on a clean eating diet is not hard or complicated. It just requires that you eat a lot of real foods and cut out the processed foods and sugar-packed beverages. But if there's one thing most people struggle with when it comes to dieting and meal-prepping, it's knowing what foods to eat and which foods are safe to eat on a clean eating diet. That's where we come in.

With our meal prep service, you don't have to worry about what you're eating. With our convenience delivered daily, you can easily eat real foods with straightforward meal plans listed at easy-to-read calorie amounts. We help you stay on track with our in-depth tracking system so that you know exactly how much protein, fat, carbs and fiber you're getting at every meal.

With clean eating meal prep meal prep, you can be as healthy as possible without having to think too hard about what to eat or when to eat. All you have to do is stop by our retail store or ship us your order for free and get ready for a healthy lifestyle!

Squash Spaghetti with Bolognese Sauce

Preparation Time: 5 minutes
Cooking Time: 10 minutes
Servings: 3
Ingredients:
1. 1 large Squash, cut into 2 and seed pulp removed
2. 2 cups Water
3. Bolognese Sauce to serve

Directions:
- Place the trivet and add the water. Add in the squash, seal the lid, select Manual and cook on High Pressure for 8 minutes. Once ready, quickly release the pressure. Carefully remove the squash; use two forks to shred the inner skin. Serve with bolognese sauce.

Nutrition: Calories 37, Protein 0.9g, Net Carbs 7.8g, Fat 0.4g

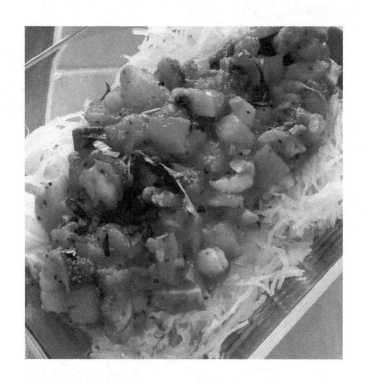

Healthy Halibut Fillets

Preparation Time: 5 minutes
Cooking Time: 10 minutes
Servings: 2
Ingredients:
1. 2 Halibut fillets
2. 1 tbsp. Dill
3. 1 tbsp. Onion powder
4. 1 cup Parsley, chopped
5. 2 tbsp. Paprika
6. 1 tbsp. Garlic powder
7. 1 tbsp. Lemon Pepper
8. 2 tbsp. Lemon juice

Directions:
- Mix lemon juice, lemon pepper, garlic powder, and paprika, parsley, dill and onion powder in a bowl. Pour the mixture in the Instant pot and place the halibut fish over it.
- Seal the lid, press Manual mode and cook for 10 minutes on High pressure. When ready, do a quick pressure release by setting the valve to venting.

Nutrition: Calories 283, Protein 22.5g, Net Carbs 6.2g, Fat 16.4g

Clean Salmon with Soy Sauce

Preparation Time: 10 minutes
Cooking Time: 30 minutes
Servings: 2
Ingredients:
1. 2 Salmon fillets
2. 2 tbsp. Avocado oil
3. 2 tbsp. Soy sauce
4. 1 tbsp. Garlic powder
5. 1 tbsp. fresh Dill to garnish
6. Salt and Pepper, to taste

Directions:
- To make the marinade, thoroughly mix the soy sauce, avocado oil, salt, pepper and garlic powder into a bowl. Dip salmon in the mixture and place in the refrigerator for 20 minutes.
- Transfer the contents to the Instant pot. Seal, set on Manual and cook for 10 minutes on high pressure. When ready, do a quick release. Serve topped with the fresh dill.

Nutrition: Calories 512, Protein 65g, Net Carbs 3.2g, Fat 21g

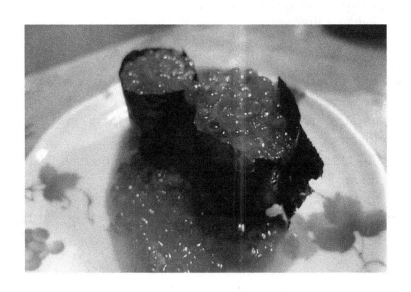

Simple Salmon with Eggs

Preparation Time: 2 minutes
Cooking Time: 5 minutes
Servings: 3
Ingredients:
1. 1 lb Salmon, cooked, mashed
2. 2 Eggs, whisked
3. 2 Onions, chopped
4. 2 stalks celery, chopped
5. 1 cup Parsley, chopped
6. 1 tbsp. Olive oil
7. Salt and Pepper, to taste

Directions:
- Mix salmon, onion, celery, parsley, and salt and pepper, in a bowl. Form into 6 patties about 1 inch thick and dip them in the whisked eggs. Heat oil in the Instant pot on Sauté mode.
- Add the patties to the pot and cook on both sides, for about 5 minutes and transfer to the plate. Allow to cool and serve.

Nutrition: Calories 331, Protein 38g, Net Carbs 5.3g, Fat 16g

Easy Shrimp

Preparation Time: 4 minutes
Cooking Time: 5 minutes
Servings: 2
Ingredients:
1. 1 lb Shrimp, peeled and deveined
2. 2 Garlic cloves, crushed
3. 1 tbsp. Butter.
4. A pinch of red Pepper
5. Salt and Pepper, to taste
6. 1 cup Parsley, chopped

Directions:
- Melt butter on Sauté mode. Add shrimp, garlic, red pepper, salt and pepper. Cook for 5 minutes, stirring occasionally the shrimp until pink. Serve topped with parsley.

Nutrition: Calories 245, Protein 45g, Net Carbs 4.8g, Fat 4g

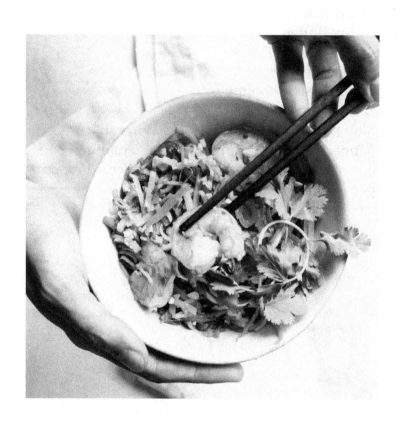

Scallops with Mushroom Special

Preparation Time: 15 minutes
Cooking Time: 20 minutes
Servings: 2
Ingredients:
1. 1 lb Scallops
2. 2 Onions, chopped
3. 1 tbsp. Butter
4. 2 tbsp. Olive oil
5. 1 cup Mushrooms
6. Salt and Pepper, to taste
7. 1 tbsp. Lemon juice
8. ½ cup Whipping Cream
9. 1 tbsp. chopped fresh Parsley

Directions:
- Heat the oil on Sauté. Add onions, butter, mushrooms, salt and pepper. Cook for 3 to 5 minutes. Add the lemon juice and scallops. Lock the lid and set to Manual mode.
- Cook for 15 minutes on High pressure. When ready, do a quick pressure release and carefully open the lid. Top with a drizzle of cream and fresh parsley.

Nutrition: Calories 312, Protein 31g, Net Carbs 7.3g, Fat 10.4g

Delicious Creamy Crab Meat

Preparation Time: 5 minutes
Cooking Time: 10 minutes
Servings: 3
Ingredients:
1. 1 lb Crab meat
2. ½ cup Cream cheese
3. 2 tbsp. Mayonnaise
4. Salt and Pepper, to taste
5. 1 tbsp. Lemon juice
6. 1 cup Cheddar cheese, shredded

Directions:
- Mix mayo, cream cheese, salt and pepper, and lemon juice in a bowl. Add in crab meat and make small balls. Place the balls inside the pot. Seal the lid and press Manual.
- Cook for 10 minutes on High pressure. When done, allow the pressure to release naturally for 10 minutes. Sprinkle the cheese over and serve!

Nutrition: Calories 443, Protein 41g, Net Carbs 2.5g, Fat 30.4g

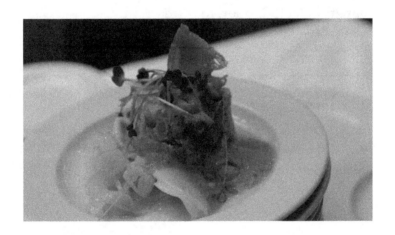

Creamy Broccoli Stew

Preparation Time: 10 minutes
Cooking Time: 20 minutes
Servings: 4
Ingredients:
1. 1 cup Heavy Cream
2. 3 oz. Parmesan cheese
3. 1 cup Broccoli florets
4. 2 Carrots, sliced
5. ½ tbsp. Garlic paste
6. ¼ tbsp. Turmeric powder
7. Salt and black Pepper, to taste
8. ½ cup Vegetable broth
9. 2 tbsp. Butter

Directions:
- Melt butter on Sauté mode. Add garlic and sauté for 30 seconds. Add broccoli and carrots, and cook until soft, for 2-3 minutes. Season with salt and pepper.
- Stir in the vegetable broth and seal the lid. Cook on Meat/Stew mode for 40 minutes. When ready, do a quick pressure release. Stir in the heavy cream.

Nutrition: Calories 239, Protein 8g, Net Carbs 5.1g, Fat 21.4g

No Crust Tomato and Spinach Quiche

Preparation Time: 10 minutes
Cooking Time: 30 minutes
Servings: 3
Ingredients:
1. 14 large Eggs
2. 1 cup Full Milk
3. Salt to taste
4. Ground Black Pepper to taste
5. 4 cups fresh Baby Spinach, chopped
6. 3 Tomatoes, diced
7. 3 Scallions, sliced
8. 2 Tomato, sliced into firm rings
9. ½ cup Parmesan Cheese, shredded
10. Water for boiling

Directions:
- Place the trivet in the pot and pour in 1 ½ cups of water. Break the eggs into a bowl, add salt, pepper, and milk and whisk it. Share the diced tomatoes, spinach and scallions into 3 ramekins, gently stir, and arrange 3 slices of tomatoes on top in each ramekin.
- Sprinkle with Parmesan cheese. Gently place the ramekins in the pot, and seal the lid. Select Manual and cook on High Pressure for 20 minutes. Once ready, quickly release the pressure.
- Carefully remove the ramekins and use a paper towel to tap soak any water from the steam that sits on the quiche. Brown the top of the quiche with a fire torch.

Nutrition: Calories 310, Protein 12g, Net Carbs 0g, Fat 27g

Peas Soup

Preparation Time: 10 minutes
Cooking Time: 10 minutes
Servings: 4
Ingredients:
1. 1 white onion, chopped
2. 1 tablespoon olive oil
3. 1 quart veggie stock
4. 2 eggs
5. 3 tablespoons lemon juice
6. 2 cups peas
7. 2 tablespoons parmesan, grated
8. Salt and black pepper to the taste

Directions:
- Heat up a pot with the oil over medium-high heat, add the onion and sauté for 4 minutes.
- Add the rest of the ingredients except the eggs, bring to a simmer and cook for 4 minutes.
- Add whisked eggs, stir the soup, cook for 2 minutes more, divide into bowls and serve.

Nutrition: Calories 293, fat 11.2 fiber 3.4, carbs 27, protein 4.45

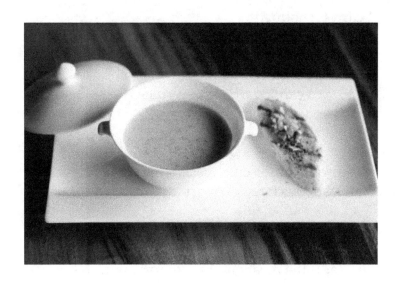

Minty Lamb Stew

Preparation Time: 10 minutes
Cooking Time: 1 hour and 45 minutes
Servings: 4
Ingredients:
1. 3 cups orange juice
2. ½ cup mint, chopped
3. Salt and black pepper to the taste
4. 2 pounds lamb shoulder, boneless and cubed
5. 3 tablespoons olive oil
6. 1 carrot, chopped
7. 1 yellow onion, chopped
8. 1 celery rib, chopped
9. 1 tablespoon ginger, grated
10. 28 ounces canned tomatoes, crushed
11. 1 tablespoon garlic, minced
12. 1 cup apricots, dried and halved
13. ½ cup mint, chopped
14. 15 ounces canned chickpeas, drained
15. 6 tablespoons Greek yogurt

Directions:
- Heat up a pot with 2 tablespoons oil over medium-high heat, add the meat and brown for 5 minutes.
- Add the carrot, onion, celery, garlic and the ginger, stir and sauté for 5 minutes more.
- Add the rest of the ingredients except the yogurt, bring to a simmer and cook over medium heat for 1 hour and 30 minutes.
- Divide the stew into bowls, top each serving with the yogurt and serve.

Nutrition: Calories 355, fat 14.3, fiber 6.7, carbs 22.6, protein 15.4

Ratatouille

Preparation Time: 5 minutes
Cooking Time: 15 minutes
Servings: 4
Ingredients:
1. 1 cup Water
2. 3 tbsp. Olive oil
3. 2 Zucchinis, sliced in rings
4. 2 Eggplants, sliced in rings
5. 3 large Tomatoes, sliced in thick rings
6. 1 medium Red Onion, sliced in thin rings
7. 3 cloves Garlic, minced
8. 2 sprigs Fresh Thyme
9. Salt to taste
10. Black Pepper to taste
11. 4 tsp Plain Vinegar

Directions:
- Place all veggies in a bowl, sprinkle with salt and pepper; toss. Line foil in a spring form tin and arrange 1 slice each of the vegetables in, one after the other in a tight circular arrangement.
- Fill the entire tin. Sprinkle the garlic over, some more black pepper and salt, and arrange the thyme sprigs on top. Drizzle olive oil and vinegar over the veggies.
- Place a trivet to fit in the Instant Pot, pour the water in and place the veggies on the trivet. Seal the lid, secure the pressure valve and select Manual mode on High Pressure for 6 minutes. Once ready, quickly release the pressure. Carefully remove the tin and serve ratatouille.

Nutrition: Calories 152, Protein 2g, Net Carbs 4g, Fat 12g

Steamed Artichokes

Preparation Time: 5 minutes
Cooking Time: 20 minutes
Servings: 3
Ingredients:
1. 2 medium Artichokes
2. 3 Lemon Wedges (for cooking and serving)
3. 1 ½ cup Water

Directions:
- Clean the artichokes by removing all dead leaves, the stem, and top third of it. Rub the top of the artichokes with the lemon. Set aside. Place a trivet to fit in the Instant Pot, pour in water.
- Place the artichokes on the trivet, seal the lid. Select Manual mode on High Pressure for 9 minutes. Once the timer ends, keep the pressure valve for 10 minutes; then quickly release the remaining pressure. Remove artichokes and serve with garlic mayo and lemon wedges.

Nutrition: Calories 47, Protein 3.3g, Net Carbs 6g, Fat 0.2g

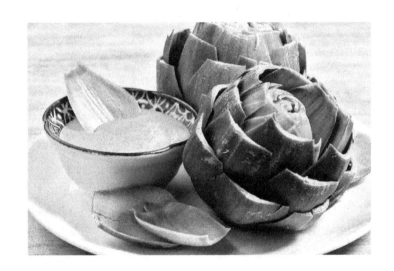

Creamed Savoy Cabbage

Preparation Time: 5 minutes
Cooking Time: 15 minutes
Servings: 3
Ingredients:
1. 2 medium Savoy Cabbages, finely chopped
2. 2 small Onions, chopped
3. 2 cups Bacon, chopped
4. 2 ½ cups Mixed Bone Broth, see recipe above
5. ¼ tsp Mace
6. 2 cups Coconut Milk
7. 1 Bay Leaf
8. Salt to taste
9. 3 tbsp. Chopped Parsley

Directions:
- Set on Sauté. Add the bacon crumbles and onions; cook until crispy. Add bone broth and scrape the bottom of the pot. Stir in bay leaf and cabbage. Cut out some parchment paper and cover the cabbage with it.
- Seal the lid, select Manual mode and cook on High Pressure for 4 minutes. Once ready, press Cancel and quickly release the pressure. Select Sauteé, stir in the milk and nutmeg. Simmer for 5 minutes, add the parsley.

Nutrition: Calories 27, Protein 4g, Net Carbs 3.1g, Fat 3g

Tilapia Delight

Preparation Time: 6 minutes
Cooking Time: 10 minutes
Servings: 4
Ingredients:
1. 4 Tilapia fillets
2. 4 tbsp. Lemon juice
3. 2 tbsp. Butter
4. 2 Garlic cloves
5. ½ cup Parsley
6. Salt and Pepper, to taste

Directions:
- Melt butter on Sauté, and add garlic cloves, parsley. Season with salt and pepper; stir well. Cook for 2 to 3 minutes. Then, add tilapia and lemon juice and stir well.
- Seal the lid and set on Manual mode. Cook for 10 minutes on High pressure. When the timer beeps, allow the pressure to release naturally, for 5 minutes.

Nutrition: Calories 135, Protein 23.7g, Net Carbs 1.3g, Fat 4.4g

Spinach Tomatoes Mix

Preparation Time: 4 minutes
Cooking Time: 10 minutes
Servings: 2
Ingredients:
1. 2 tbsp. Butter
2. 1 Onion, chopped
3. 2 cloves Garlic, minced
4. 1 tbsp. Cumin powder
5. 1 tbsp. Paprika
6. 2 Tomatoes, chopped
7. 2 cups Vegetable broth
8. 1 small bunch of Spinach, chopped
9. Cilantro for garnishing

Directions:
- Melt the butter on Sauté mode. Add onion, garlic, and cumin powder, paprika, and vegetable broth; stir well. Add in tomatoes and spinach. Seal the lid, press Manual and cook on High pressure for 10 minutes. When ready, do a quick pressure release.

Nutrition: Calories 125, Protein 7.7g, Net Carbs 8.3g, Fat 5.5g

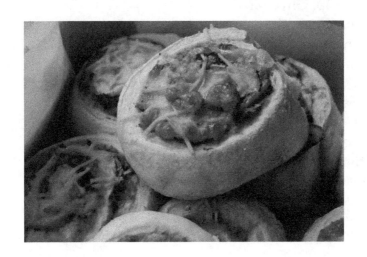

Spinach Almond Tortilla

Preparation Time: 5 minutes
Cooking Time: 10 minutes
Servings: 3
Ingredients:
1. 1 cup Almond flour + extra for dusting
2. 1 cup Spinach, chopped
3. ¼ tbsp. Chili flakes
4. ¼ cup Mushrooms, sliced
5. ½ tbsp. Salt
6. 2 tbsp. Olive oil

Directions:
- In a bowl, combine flour, mushrooms, spinach, salt, and flakes; mix well. Add ¼ cup of water and make a thick batter. Roll out the batter until is thin. Heat oil on Sauté mode.
- Cook the tortilla for 5 minutes until golden brown. Serve with cilantro sauce and enjoy.

Nutrition: Calories 165, Protein 5g, Net Carbs 2.1g, Fat 9g

Zucchini Noodles in Garlic and Parmesan Toss

Preparation Time: 5 minutes
Cooking Time: 15 minutes
Servings: 4
Ingredients:
1. 3 large Zucchinis, spiralized
2. 2 tbsp. Olive oil
3. 3 cloves Garlic, minced
4. 1 Lemon, zested and juiced
5. Salt to taste
6. Black Pepper to taste
7. 5 Mint Leaves, chopped
8. 6 tbsp. Parmesan Cheese, grated

Directions:
- Set on Sauté. Heat the oil, and add lemon zest, garlic, and salt. Stir and cook for 30 seconds. Add zucchini and pour lemon juice over. Coat the noodles quickly but gently with the oil.
- Cook for 10 seconds, press Cancel. Sprinkle the mint leaves and cheese over and toss gently.

Nutrition: Calories 15, Protein 10g, Net Carbs 2g, Fat 2g

Lemoned Broccoli

Preparation Time: 5 minutes
Cooking Time: 10 minutes
Servings: 3
Ingredients:
1. 1 lb Broccoli, cut in biteable sizes
2. 3 Lemon Slices
3. ¼ cup Water
4. Salt to taste
5. Pepper to taste

Directions:
- Pour the water into the Instant Pot. Add the broccoli and sprinkle with lemon juice, pepper, and salt. Seal the lid, secure the pressure valve, and Manual in Low Pressure mode for 3 minutes. Once ready, quickly release the pressure. Drain the broccoli and serve as a side dish.

Nutrition: Calories 34, Protein 2.8g, Net Carbs 5.6g, Fat 0.4g

Beets with Yogurt

Preparation Time: 10 minutes
Cooking Time: 40 minutes
Servings: 3 to 4
Ingredients:
1. 1 lb Beets, washed
2. 1 Lime, zested and juiced
3. 1 cup Plain Full Milk Yogurt
4. 1 clove Garlic, minced
5. Salt to taste
6. 1 tbsp. Fresh Dill, chopped
7. 1 tbsp. Olive oil to drizzle
8. Black Pepper to garnish
9. 1 cup Water

Directions:
- Pour the water in the Instant Pot and fit in a steamer basket. Add the beets, seal the lid, secure the pressure valve and select Manual mode on High Pressure mode for 30 minutes.
- Once ready, do a natural pressure release for 10 minutes, then quickly release the remaining pressure. Remove the beets to a bowl to cool, and then remove the skin. Cut into wedges.
- Place beets in a dip plate, drizzle the olive oil and lime juice over; set aside. In a bowl, mix garlic, yogurt and lime zest. Pour over the beets and garnish with black pepper, salt, and dill.

Nutrition: Calories 102, Protein 5.7g, Net Carbs 8.2g, Fat 3.8g

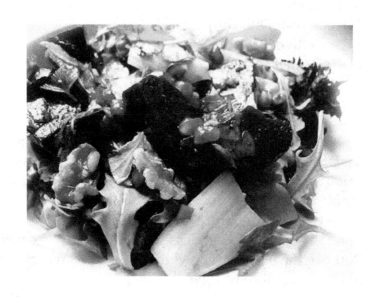

Vegetarian Faux Stew

Preparation Time: 5 minutes
Cooking Time: 25 minutes
Servings: 3
Ingredients:
1. 1 ½ cups Diced Tomatoes
2. 4 cloves Garlic
3. 1 tsp Minced Ginger
4. 1 tsp Turmeric
5. 1 tsp Cayenne Powder
6. 2 tsp Paprika
7. Salt to taste
8. 1 tsp Cumin Powder
9. 2 cups Dry Soy Curls
10. 1 ½ cups Water
11. 3 tbsp. Butter
12. ½ cup Heavy Cream
13. ¼ cup Chopped Cilantro

Directions:
- Place the tomatoes, water, soy curls and all spices in the Instant Pot. Seal the lid, secure the pressure valve and select Manual mode on High Pressure mode for 6 minutes.
- Once ready, do a natural pressure release for 10 minutes. Select Sauté, add the cream and butter. Stir while crushing the tomatoes with the back of the spoon. Stir in the cilantro and serve.

Nutrition: Calories 143, Protein 4g, Net Carbs 2g, Fat 9g

Vegetable en Papillote

Preparation Time: 5 minutes
Cooking Time: 15 minutes
Servings: 3
Ingredients:
1. 1 cup Green Beans
2. 4 small Carrots, widely julienned
3. ¼ tsp Black Pepper
4. A pinches Salt
5. 1 clove Garlic, crushed
6. 2 tbsp. Butter
7. 2 slices Lemon
8. 1 tbsp. Chopped Thyme
9. 1 tbsp. Oregano
10. 1 tbsp. Chopped Parsley
11. 17 inch Parchment Paper

Directions:
- Add all ingredients, except lemon slices and butter, in a bowl and toss. Place the paper on a flat surface and add the mixed ingredients at the center of the paper. Put the lemon slices on top and drop the butter over. Wrap it up well.
- Pour 1 cup of water in and lower the trivet with handle. Put the veggie pack on the trivet, seal the lid, and cook on High Pressure for 2 minutes. Once ready, do a quick release. Carefully remove the packet and serve veggies in a wrap on a plate.

Nutrition: Calories 60, Protein 3g, Net Carbs 1g, Fat 3g

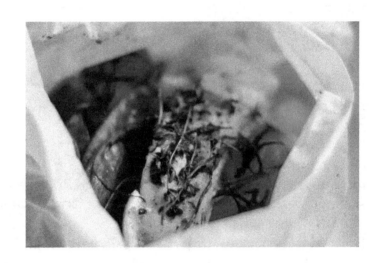

Faux Beet Risotto

Preparation Time: 5 minutes
Cooking Time: 15 minutes
Servings: 2
Ingredients:
1. 4 Beets, tails and leafs removed
2. 2 tbsp. Olive oil
3. 1 big head Cauliflower, cut into florets
4. 4 tbsp. cup Full Milk
5. 2 tsp Red Chili Flakes
6. Salt to taste
7. Black Pepper to taste
8. ½ cup Water

Directions:
- Pour the water in the Instant Pot and fit a steamer basket. Place the beets and cauliflower in the basket. Seal the lid, and cook on High Pressure mode for 4 minutes.
- Once ready, do a natural pressure release for 10 minutes, then quickly release the pressure.Remove the steamer basket with the vegetables and discard water. Remove the beets' peels.
- Place veggies back to the pot, add salt, pepper, and flakes. Mash with a potato masher. Hit Sauté, and cook the milk for 2 minutes. Stir frequently. Dish onto plates and drizzle with oil.

Nutrition: Calories 153, Protein 3.6g, Net Carbs 2.5g, Fat 9g

Broccoli Rice with Mushrooms

Preparation Time: 5 minutes
Cooking Time: 30 minutes
Servings: 3
Ingredients:
1. 2 tbsp. Olive oil
2. 1 small Red Onion, chopped
3. 1 Carrot, chopped
4. 2 cups Button Mushrooms, chopped
5. ½ Lemon, zested and juiced
6. Salt to taste
7. Pepper to taste
8. 2 cloves Garlic, minced
9. ½ cup Broccoli rice
10. ½ cup Chicken Stock
11. 5 Cherry Tomatoes
12. Parsley Leaves, chopped for garnishing

Directions:
- Set on Sauté. Heat oil, and cook the carrots and onions for 2 minutes. Stir in mushrooms, and cook for 3 minutes. Stir in pepper, salt, lemon juice, garlic, and lemon zest.
- Stir in broccoli and chicken stock. Drop the tomatoes over the top, but don't stir. Seal the lid, and cook on High pressure for 10 minutes. Once ready, do a natural pressure release for 4 minutes, then quickly release the remaining pressure. Sprinkle with parsley and stir evenly.

Nutrition: Calories 160, Protein 6g, Net Carbs 10g, Fat 2g

Sides

Parmesan Roasted Broccoli

Preparation Time: 10 minutes
Cooking Time: 20 minutes
Servings: 6
Ingredients:
1. 3 tablespoons of olive oil
2. 4 cups of broccoli florets
3. 3 tablespoons of vegan parmesan, grated
4. ½ teaspoon of Italian seasoning
5. 1 tablespoon of lemon juice
6. 1 tablespoon parsley, chopped
7. Pepper and salt to taste

Directions:
- Preheat your oven to 450 degrees F. Apply cooking spray on your pan.
- Keep the broccoli florets in a freezer bag.
- Now add the Italian seasoning, olive oil, pepper, and salt.
- Seal your bag. Shake it. Coat well.
- Pour your broccoli on the pan. It should be in one layer.
- Bake for 20 minutes. Stir halfway through.
- Take out from your oven. Sprinkle parsley and parmesan.
- Drizzle some lemon juice.
- You can garnish with lemon wedges if you want.

Nutrition:
Calories 96
Carbohydrates 4g
Cholesterol 2mg

Total Fat 8g
Protein 2g
Sugar 1g
Fiber 1g
Sodium 58mg
Potassium 191mg

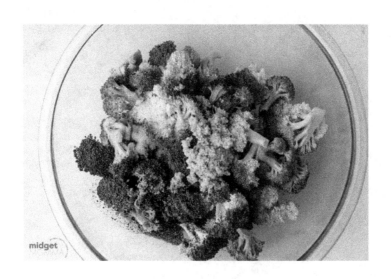

Thyme with Honey-Roasted Carrots

Preparation Time: 5 minutes
Cooking Time: 30 minutes
Servings: 4
Ingredients:
1. 1/5 lb. carrots, with the tops
2. 1 tablespoon of honey
3. 2 tablespoons of olive oil
4. ½ teaspoon thyme, dried
5. ½ teaspoon of sea salt

Directions:
- Preheat your oven to 425 degrees F.
- Keep parchment paper on your baking sheet.
- Toss your carrots with honey, oil, thyme, and salt. Coat well.
- Keep in a single layer. Bake in your oven for 30 minutes.
- Set aside for cooling before serving.

Nutrition:
Calories 85
Carbohydrates 6g
Cholesterol 0mg
Total Fat 8g
Protein 1g
Sugar 6g
Fiber 1g
Sodium 244mg

Roasted Parsnips

Preparation Time: 5 minutes
Cooking Time: 30 minutes
Servings: 4
Ingredients:
1. 1 tablespoon of extra-virgin olive oil
2. 2 lbs. parsnips
3. 1 teaspoon of kosher salt
4. 1-1/2 teaspoon of Italian seasoning
5. Chopped parsley for garnishing

Directions:
- Preheat your oven to 400 degrees F.
- Peel the parsnips. Cut them into one-inch chunks.
- Now toss with the seasoning, salt, and oil in a bowl.
- Spread this on your baking sheet. It should be in one layer.
- Roast for 30 minutes. Stir every ten minutes.
- Transfer to a plate. Garnish with parsley.

Nutrition:
Calories 124
Carbohydrates 20g
Total Fat 4g
Protein 2g
Fiber 4g
Sugar 5g
Sodium 550mg

Green Beans

Preparation Time: 5 minutes
Cooking Time: 10 minutes
Servings: 5
Ingredients:
1. ½ teaspoon of red pepper flakes
2. 2 tablespoons of extra-virgin olive oil
3. 2 garlic cloves, minced
4. 1-1/2 lbs. green beans, trimmed
5. 2 tablespoons of water
6. ½ teaspoon kosher salt

Directions:
- Heat oil in a skillet on medium temperature.
- Include the pepper flake. Stir to coat in the olive oil.
- Include the green beans. Cook for 7 minutes.
- Stir often. The beans should be brown in some areas.
- Add the salt and garlic. Cook for 1 minute, while stirring.
- Pour water and cover immediately.
- Cook covered for 1 more minute.

Nutrition:
Calories 82
Carbohydrates 6g
Total Fat 6g
Protein 1g
Fiber 2g
Sugar 0g
Sodium 230mg

Roasted Carrots

Preparation Time: 10 minutes
Cooking Time: 40 minutes
Servings: 4
Ingredients:
1. 1 onion, peeled & cut
2. 8 carrots, peeled & cut
3. 1 teaspoon thyme, chopped
4. 2 tablespoons of extra-virgin olive oil
5. ½ teaspoon rosemary, chopped
6. ¼ teaspoon ground pepper
7. ½ teaspoon salt

Directions:
- Preheat your oven to 425 degrees F.
- Mix the onions and carrots by tossing in a bowl with rosemary, thyme, pepper, and salt. Spread on your baking sheet.
- Roast for 40 minutes. The onions and carrots should be browning and tender.

Nutrition:
Calories 126
Carbohydrates 16g
Total Fat 6g
Protein 2g
Fiber 4g
Sugar 8g
Sodium 286mg

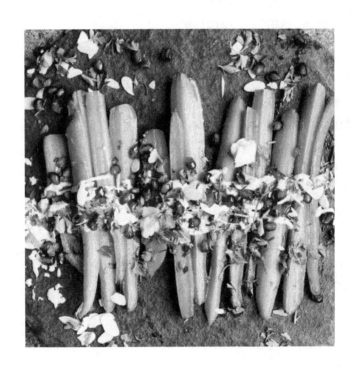

Tomato Bulgur

Preparation Time: 7 minutes
Cooking Time: 20 minutes
Servings: 2
Ingredients:
1. ½ cup bulgur
2. 1 teaspoon tomato paste
3. ½ white onion, diced
4. 2 tablespoons coconut oil
5. 1 ½ cup chicken stock

Directions:
- Toss coconut oil in the pan and melt it.
- Add diced onion and roast it until light brown.
- Then add bulgur and stir well.
- Cook bulgur in coconut oil for 3 minutes.
- Then add tomato paste and mix up bulgur until homogenous.
- Add chicken stock.
- Close the lid and cook bulgur for 15 minutes over the medium heat.
- The cooked bulgur should soak all liquid.

Nutrition:
Calories 257
Fat 14.5
Fiber 7.1
Carbs 30.2
Protein 5.2

Moroccan Style Couscous

Preparation Time: 10 minutes
Cooking Time: 10 minutes
Servings: 4
Ingredients:
1. 1 cup yellow couscous
2. ½ teaspoon ground cardamom
3. 1 cup chicken stock
4. 1 tablespoon butter
5. 1 teaspoon salt
6. ½ teaspoon red pepper

Directions:
- Toss butter in the pan and melt it.
- Add couscous and roast it for 1 minute over the high heat.
- Then add ground cardamom, salt, and red pepper. Stir it well.
- Pour the chicken stock and bring the mixture to boil.
- Simmer couscous for 5 minutes with the closed lid.

Nutrition:
Calories 196
Fat 3.4
Fiber 2.4
Carbs 35
Protein 5.9

Creamy Polenta

Preparation Time: 8 minutes
Cooking Time: 45 minutes
Servings: 4
Ingredients:
1. 1 cup polenta
2. 1 ½ cup water
3. 2 cups chicken stock
4. ½ cup cream
5. 1/3 cup Parmesan, grated

Directions:
- Put polenta in the pot.
- Add water, chicken stock, cream, and Parmesan. Mix up polenta well.
- Then preheat oven to 355F.
- Cook polenta in the oven for 45 minutes.
- Mix up the cooked meal with the help of the spoon carefully before serving.

Nutrition:
Calories 208
Fat 5.3
Fiber 1
Carbs 32.2
Protein 8

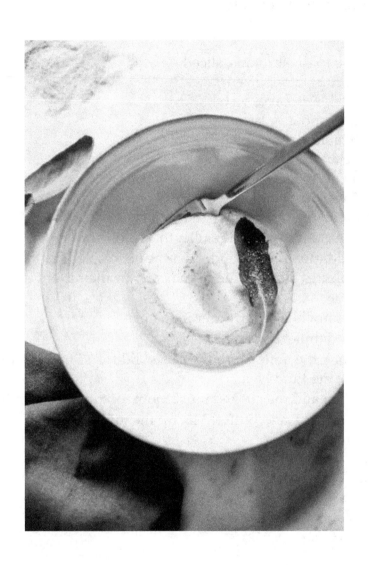

Mushroom Millet

Preparation Time: 10 minutes
Cooking Time: 15 minutes
Servings: 3
Ingredients:
1. ¼ cup mushrooms, sliced
2. ¾ cup onion, diced
3. 1 tablespoon olive oil
4. 1 teaspoon salt
5. 3 tablespoons milk
6. ½ cup millet
7. 1 cup of water
8. 1 teaspoon butter

Directions:
- Pour olive oil in the skillet then put the onion.
- Add mushrooms and roast the vegetables for 10 minutes over the medium heat. Stir them from time to time.
- Meanwhile, pour water in the pan.
- Add millet and salt.
- Cook the millet with the closed lid for 15 minutes over the medium heat.
- Then add the cooked mushroom mixture in the millet.
- Add milk and butter. Mix up the millet well.

Nutrition:
Calories 198
Fat 7.7
Fiber 3.5
Carbs 27.9
Protein 4.7

Spicy Barley

Preparation Time: 7 minutes
Cooking Time: 42 minutes
Servings: 5
Ingredients:
1. 1 cup barley
2. 3 cups chicken stock
3. ½ teaspoon cayenne pepper
4. 1 teaspoon salt
5. ½ teaspoon chili pepper
6. ½ teaspoon ground black pepper
7. 1 teaspoon butter
8. 1 teaspoon olive oil

Directions:
- Place barley and olive oil in the pan.
- Roast barley on high heat for 1 minute. Stir it well.
- Then add salt, chili pepper, ground black pepper, cayenne pepper, and butter.
- Add chicken stock.
- Close the lid and cook barley for 40 minutes over the medium-low heat.

Nutrition:
Calories 152
Fat 2.9
Fiber 6.5
Carbs 27.8
Protein 5.1

Tender Farro

Preparation Time: 8 minutes
Cooking Time: 40 minutes
Servings: 4
Ingredients:
1. 1 cup farro
2. 3 cups beef broth
3. 1 teaspoon salt
4. 1 tablespoon almond butter
5. 1 tablespoon dried dill

Directions:
- Place farro in the pan.
- Add beef broth, dried dill, and salt.
- Close the lid and place the mixture to boil.
- Then boil it for 35 minutes over the medium-low heat.
- When the time is done, open the lid and add almond butter.
- Mix up the cooked farro well.

Nutrition:
Calories 95
Fat 3.3
Fiber 1.3
Carbs 10.1
Protein 6.4

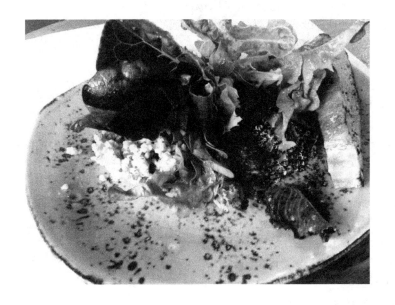

Wheatberry Salad

Preparation Time: 10 minutes
Cooking Time: 50 minutes
Servings: 2
Ingredients:
1. ¼ cup of wheat berries
2. 1 cup of water
3. 1 teaspoon salt
4. 2 tablespoons walnuts, chopped
5. 1 tablespoon chives, chopped
6. ¼ cup fresh parsley, chopped
7. 2 oz. pomegranate seeds
8. 1 tablespoon canola oil
9. 1 teaspoon chili flakes

Directions:
- Place wheat berries and water in the pan.
- Add salt and simmer the ingredients for 50 minutes over the medium heat.
- Meanwhile, mix up together walnuts, chives, parsley, pomegranate seeds, and chili flakes.
- When the wheatberry is cooked, transfer it in the walnut mixture.
- Add canola oil and mix up the salad well.

Nutrition:
Calories 160
Fat 11.8
Fiber 1.2
Carbs 12
Protein 3.4

Curry Wheatberry Rice

Preparation Time: 10 minutes
Cooking Time: 1 hour 15 minutes
Servings: 5
Ingredients:
1. 1 tablespoon curry paste
2. ¼ cup milk
3. 1 cup wheat berries
4. ½ cup of rice
5. 1 teaspoon salt
6. 4 tablespoons olive oil
7. 6 cups chicken stock

Directions:
- Place wheatberries and chicken stock in the pan.
- Close the lid and cook the mixture for 1 hour over the medium heat.
- Then add rice, olive oil, and salt.
- Stir well.
- Mix up together milk and curry paste.
- Add the curry liquid in the rice-wheatberry mixture and stir well.
- Boil the meal for 15 minutes with the closed lid.
- When the rice is cooked, all the meal is cooked.

Nutrition:
Calories 232
Fat 15
Fiber 1.4
Carbs 23.5
Protein 3.9

Couscous Salad

Preparation Time: 10 minutes
Cooking Time: 6 minutes
Servings: 4
Ingredients:
1. 1/3 cup couscous
2. 1/3 cup chicken stock
3. ¼ teaspoon ground black pepper
4. ¾ teaspoon ground coriander
5. ½ teaspoon salt
6. ¼ teaspoon paprika
7. ¼ teaspoon turmeric
8. 1 tablespoon butter
9. 2 oz. chickpeas, canned, drained
10. 1 cup fresh arugula, chopped
11. 2 oz. sun-dried tomatoes, chopped
12. 1 oz. Feta cheese, crumbled
13. 1 tablespoon canola oil

Directions:
- Bring the chicken stock to boil.
- Add couscous, ground black pepper, ground coriander, salt, paprika, and turmeric. Add chickpeas and butter. Stir the mixture well and close the lid.
- Let the couscous soak the hot chicken stock for 6 minutes.
- Meanwhile, in the mixing bowl combine together arugula, sun-dried tomatoes, and Feta cheese.
- Add cooked couscous mixture and canola oil.
- Mix up the salad well.

Nutrition:
Calories 18
Fat 9
Fiber 3.6
Carbs 21.1
Protein 6

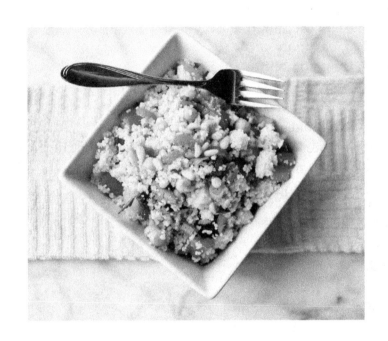

Citrus Couscous with Herb

Preparation Time: 5 minutes
Cooking Time: 15 minutes
Servings: 2
Ingredients:
1. 1/3 cup couscous
2. ¼ cup of water
3. 4 tablespoons orange juice
4. ¼ orange, chopped
5. 1 teaspoon Italian seasonings
6. 1/3 teaspoon salt
7. ½ teaspoon butter

Directions:
- Pour water and orange juice in the pan.
- Add orange, Italian seasoning, and salt.
- Bring the liquid to boil and remove it from the heat.
- Add butter and couscous. Stir well and close the lid.
- Leave the couscous rest for 10 minutes.

Nutrition:
Calories 149,
Fat 1.9
Fiber 2.1
Carbs 28.5
 Protein 4.1

Mascarpone Couscous

Preparation Time: 15 minutes
Cooking Time: 7.5 hours
Servings: 4
Ingredients:
1. 1 cup couscous
2. 3 ½ cup chicken stock
3. ½ cup mascarpone
4. 1 teaspoon salt
5. 1 teaspoon ground paprika

Directions:
- Place chicken stock and mascarpone in the pan and bring the liquid to boil.
- Add salt and ground paprika. Stir gently and simmer for 1 minute.
- Take off the liquid from the heat and add couscous. Stir well and close the lid.
- Leave couscous for 10 minutes.
- Stir the cooked side dish well before serving.

Nutrition:
Calories 227
Fat 4.9
Fiber 2.4
Carbs 35.4
Protein 9.7

Crispy Corn

Preparation Time: 8 minutes
Cooking Time: 5 minutes
Servings: 3
Ingredients:
1. 1 cup corn kernels
2. 1 tablespoon coconut flour
3. ½ teaspoon salt
4. 3 tablespoons canola oil
5. ½ teaspoon ground paprika
6. ¾ teaspoon chili pepper
7. 1 tablespoon water

Directions:
- In the mixing bowl, combine together corn kernels with salt and coconut flour.
- Add water and mix up the corn with the help of the spoon.
- Pour canola oil in the skillet and heat it.
- Add corn kernels mixture and roast it for 4 minutes. Stir it from time to time.
- When the corn kernels are crunchy, transfer them in the plate and dry with the paper towel's help.
- Add chili pepper and ground paprika. Mix up well.

Nutrition:
Calories 179
Fat 15
Fiber 2.4
Carbs 11.3
Protein 2.1

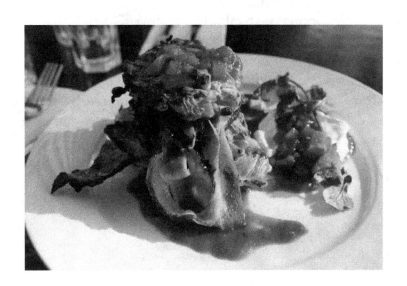

Shoepeg Corn Salad

Preparation Time: 10 minutes
Cooking Time: 0 minute
Servings: 4
Ingredients:
1. ¼ cup Greek yogurt
2. 1 cup shoepeg corn, drained
3. ½ cup cherry tomatoes halved
4. 1 jalapeno pepper, chopped
5. 1 tablespoon lemon juice
6. 3 tablespoons fresh cilantro, chopped
7. 1 tablespoon chives, chopped

Directions:
- In the salad bowl, mix up together shoepeg corn, cherry tomatoes, jalapeno pepper, chives, and fresh cilantro.
- Add lemon juice and Greek yogurt. Mix yo the salad well.
- Place in the refrigerator and store it for up to 1 day.

Nutrition:
Calories 49
Fat 0.7
Fiber 1.2
Carbs 9.4
Protein 2.7

Farro Salad with Arugula

Preparation Time: 10 minutes
Cooking Time: 35 minutes
Servings: 2
Ingredients:
1. ½ cup farro
2. 1 ½ cup chicken stock
3. 1 teaspoon salt
4. ½ teaspoon ground black pepper
5. 2 cups arugula, chopped
6. 1 cucumber, chopped
7. 1 tablespoon lemon juice
8. ½ teaspoon olive oil
9. ½ teaspoon Italian seasoning

Directions:
- Mix up together farro, salt, and chicken stock and transfer mixture in the pan.
- Close the lid and boil it for 35 minutes.
- Meanwhile, place all remaining ingredients in the salad bowl.
- Chill the farro to the room temperature and add it in the salad bowl too.
- Mix up the salad well.

Nutrition:
Calories 92
Fat 2.3
Fiber 2
Carbs 15.6
Protein 3.9

Stir-Fried Farros

Preparation Time: 5 minutes
Cooking Time: 35 minutes
Servings: 2
Ingredients:
1. ½ cup farro
2. 1 ½ cup water
3. 1 teaspoon salt
4. 1 teaspoon chili flakes
5. ½ teaspoon paprika
6. ½ teaspoon turmeric
7. ½ teaspoon ground coriander
8. 1 yellow onion, sliced
9. 1 tablespoon butter
10. 1 carrot, grated

Directions:
- Place farro in the pan. Add water and salt.
- Close the lid and boil it for 30 minutes.
- Meanwhile, toss the butter in the skillet.
- Heat it and add sliced onion and grated carrot.
- Fry the vegetables for 10 minutes over the medium heat. Stir them with the help of spatula from time to time.
- When the farro is cooked, add it in the roasted vegetables and mix up well.
- Cook stir-fried farro for 5 minutes over the medium-high heat.

Nutrition:
Calories 129
Fat 5.9
Fiber 3
Carbs 17.1
Protein 2.8

Cauliflower Broccoli Mash

Preparation Time: 5 minutes
Cooking Time: 10 minutes
Serving: 6
Ingredients:
1. 1 large head cauliflower, cut into chunks
2. 1 small head broccoli, cut into florets
3. 3 tablespoons extra virgin olive oil
4. 1 teaspoon salt
5. Pepper, to taste

Directions:
- Take a pot and add oil then heat it
- Add the cauliflower and broccoli
- Season with salt and pepper to taste
- Keep stirring to make vegetable soft
- Add water if needed
- When is already cooked, use a food processor or a potato masher to puree the vegetables
- Serve and enjoy!

Nutrition:
Calories: 39
Fat: 3g
Carbohydrates: 2g
Protein: 0.89g

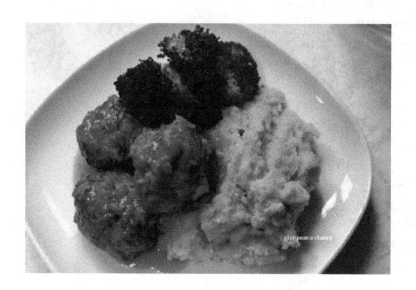

Roasted Curried Cauliflower

Preparation Time: 5 minutes
Cooking Time: 30 minutes
Serving: 4
Ingredients:
1. 1 large head cauliflower, cut into florets
2. 1 teaspoon curry powder
3. 1 and ½ tablespoon olive oil
4. 1 teaspoon cumin seeds
5. 1 teaspoon mustard seeds
6. ¾ teaspoon salt

Directions:
- Preheat your oven to 375 degrees F
- Grease a baking sheet with cooking spray
- Take a bowl and place all ingredients
- Toss to coat well
- Arrange the vegetable on a baking sheet
- Roast for 30 minutes
- Serve and enjoy!

Nutrition:
Calories: 67
Fat: 6g
Carbohydrates: 4g
Protein: 2g

Caramelized Pears and Onions

Preparation Time: 5 minutes
Cooking Time: 35 minutes
Serving: 4
Ingredients:
1. 2 red onion, cut into wedges
2. 2 firm red pears, cored and quartered
3. 1 tablespoon olive oil
4. Salt and pepper, to taste

Directions:
- Preheat your oven to 425 degrees F
- Place the pears and onion on a baking tray
- Drizzle with olive oil
- Season with salt and pepper
- Bake in the oven for 35 minutes
- Serve and enjoy!

Nutrition:
Calories: 101
Fat: 4g
Carbohydrates: 17g
Protein: 1g

Spicy Roasted Brussels Sprouts

Preparation Time: 5 minutes
Cooking Time: 30 minutes
Serving: 4
Ingredients:
1. 1 and ¼ pound Brussels sprouts, cut into florets
2. ½ cup kimchi with juice
3. 2 tablespoons olive oil
4. Salt and pepper, to taste

Directions:
- Set the oven to 425 F.
- Toss the Brussels sprouts with pepper, salt, and oil.
- Bake in the oven for 25 minutes
- Remove from oven and mix with kimchi
- Return to the oven
- Cook for 5 minutes
- Serve and enjoy!

Nutrition:
Calories: 135
Fat: 7g
Carbohydrates: 16g
Protein: 5g

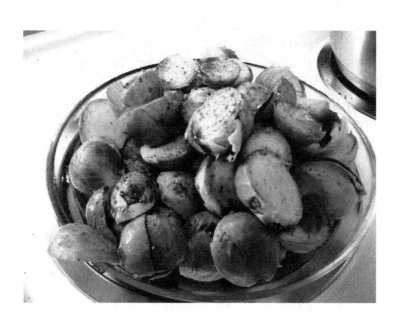

Cool Garbanzo and Spinach Beans

Preparation Time: 5-10 minutes
Cooking Time: 0 minute
Serving: 4
Ingredients:
1. 12 ounces garbanzo beans
2. 1 tablespoon olive oil
3. ½ onion, diced
4. ½ teaspoon cumin
5. 10 ounces spinach, chopped

Directions:
- Take a skillet and add olive oil
- Place it over medium-low heat
- Add onions, garbanzo and cook for 5 minutes
- Stir in cumin, garbanzo beans, spinach and season with sunflower seeds
- Use a spoon to smash gently
- Cook thoroughly
- Serve and enjoy!

Nutrition:
Calories: 90
Fat: 4g
Carbohydrates:11g
Protein:4g

Onion and Orange Healthy Salad

Preparation Time: 10 minutes
Cooking Time: 0 minutes
Serving: 3
Ingredients:
1. 6 large orange
2. 3 tablespoon of red wine vinegar
3. 6 tablespoon of olive oil
4. 1 teaspoon of dried oregano
5. 1 red onion, thinly sliced
6. 1 cup olive oil
7. ¼ cup of fresh chives, chopped
8. Ground black pepper

Directions:
- Peel the orange and cut each of them in 4-5 crosswise slices
- Transfer the oranges to a shallow dish
- Drizzle vinegar, olive oil and sprinkle oregano
- Toss
- Chill for 30 minutes
- Arrange sliced onion and black olives on top
- Decorate with an additional sprinkle of chives and a fresh grind of pepper
- Serve and enjoy!

Nutrition:
Calories: 120
Fat: 6g
Carbohydrates: 20g
Protein: 2g

Stir-Fried Almond And Spinach

Preparation Time: 10 minutes
Cooking Time: 15 minutes
Serving: 2
Ingredients:
1. 34 pounds spinach
2. 3 tablespoons almonds
3. Salt to taste
4. 1 tablespoon coconut oil

Directions:
- Put oil to a large pot and place it on high heat
- Add spinach and let it cook, stirring frequently
- Once the spinach is cooked and tender, season with salt and stir
- Add almonds and enjoy!

Nutrition:
Calories: 150
Fat: 12g
Carbohydrates: 10g
Protein: 8g

Cilantro And Avocado Platter

Preparation Time: 10 minutes
Cooking Time: 0 minutes
Serving: 6
Ingredients:
1. 2 avocados, peeled, pitted and diced
2. 1 sweet onion, chopped
3. 1 green bell pepper, chopped
4. 1 large ripe tomato, chopped
5. ¼ cup of fresh cilantro, chopped
6. ½ a lime, juiced
7. Salt and pepper as needed

Directions:
- Take a medium-sized bowl and add onion, bell pepper, tomato, avocados, lime and cilantro
- Mix well and give it a toss
- Season with salt and pepper according to your taste
- Serve and enjoy!

Nutrition:
Calories: 126
Fat: 10g
Carbohydrates: 10g
Protein: 2g

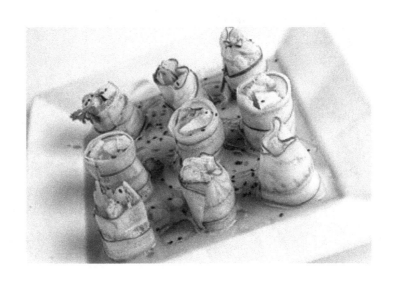

Spicy Wasabi Mayonnaise

Preparation Time: 15 minutes
Cooking Time: 0 minute
Serving: 4
Ingredients:
- ½ tablespoon wasabi paste
1. 1 cup mayonnaise

Directions:
1. Take a bowl and mix wasabi paste and mayonnaise
2. Mix well
3. Let it chill, use as needed
4. Serve and enjoy

Nutrition:
Calories: 388
Fat: 42g
Carbohydrates: 1g
Protein: 1g

Roasted Portobellos With Rosemary

Preparation Time: 5 minutes
Cooking Time: 15 minutes
Serving: 4
Ingredients:
2. 8 portobello mushroom, trimmed
3. 1 sprig rosemary, torn
4. 2 tablespoons fresh lemon juice
5. ¼ cup extra virgin olive oil
6. 1 clove garlic, minced
7. Salt and pepper, to taste

Directions:
- Preheat your oven to 450 degrees F
- Take a bowl and add all ingredients
- Toss to coat
- Place the mushroom in a baking sheet stem side up
- Roast in the oven for 15 minutes
- Serve and enjoy!

Nutrition:
Calories: 63
Fat: 6g
Carbohydrates: 2g
Protein:1g

Green, Red and Yellow Rice

Preparation Time: 5 minutes
Cooking Time: 15 minutes
Servings: 10
Ingredients:

- 2 cups brown rice, rinsed
- 2 cups green onions, chopped
- ¼ cup garlic, finely chopped
- 2 cups red bell pepper, chopped
- 2 cups frozen corn, thawed
- 2 tablespoons olive oil
- 1 cup fresh cilantro, chopped
- Salt to taste
- Pepper to taste
- Cayenne pepper to taste

Directions:

1. Place a large saucepan over medium heat. Add 4 cups water and brown rice and cook according to the instructions on the package. Once cooked, cover and set aside.
2. Place a large skillet over medium heat. Add oil. When the oil is heated, add garlic and sauté for about a minute until aromatic.
3. Add corn, red bell pepper, green onion, salt, pepper and cayenne pepper and sauté for 2-3 minutes.
4. Add rice and cilantro. Mix well and heat thoroughly.
5. Serve.

Nutrition:
Calories: 89 kcal
Protein: 2.41 g
Fat: 4.01 g
Carbohydrates: 11.26 g

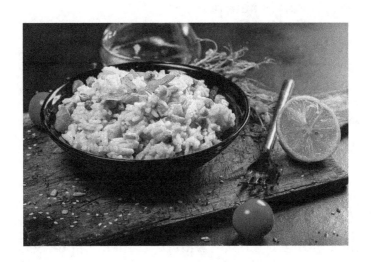

Spiced Sweet Potato Bread

Preparation Time: 15 minutes
Cooking Time: 45-55 minutes
Servings: 2
Ingredients:
For dry **Ingredients:**
1. 1 cup coconut flour
2. 2 teaspoons ground nutmeg
3. 2 tablespoons ground cinnamon
4. 1 teaspoon ground mace
5. 2 teaspoons baking powder
6. 2 teaspoons baking soda
7. ¼ teaspoon sea salt

Wet **Ingredients:**
- 4 large sweet potatoes, peeled, thinly sliced
- 8 large eggs
- 1 cup almond butter
- 2 teaspoons organic almond extract
- 8 tablespoons melted grass fed butter, unsalted
- 4 tablespoons coconut oil

Directions:
1. Grease 2 loaf pans of 9 x 5 inches with coconut oil. Line the bottom of the pan with parchment paper. Set aside.
2. Place a medium saucepan over medium heat. Add sweet potatoes. Pour enough water to cover the sweet potatoes. Cook until the sweet potatoes are tender.
3. Turn off the heat and drain the sweet potatoes.
4. Add the sweet potatoes back into the pan. Mash with a potato masher until smooth. Let it cool completely.
5. Put all together the dry ingredients into a bowl and mix well.
6. Add eggs into a large bowl and whisk well. Add sweet potatoes, butter, almond extract and almond butter and whisk until well combined.

7. Add the dry ingredients into the bowl of wet ingredients and whisk until well combined.
8. Divide the batter into the prepared loaf pans.
9. Bake in a preheated oven at 350°F for about 45 -55 minutes or a toothpick when inserted in the center of the loaf comes out clean.
10. Remove from oven and cool completely.
11. Slice with a sharp knife into slices of 1-inch thickness.

Nutrition:
Calories: 1738 kcal
Protein: 27 g
Fat: 145.92 g
Carbohydrates: 89.58 g

Broccoli and Black Beans Stir Fry

Preparation Time: 10 minutes
Cooking Time: 15 minutes
Servings: 4
Ingredients:
- 4 cups broccoli florets
- 1 tablespoon sesame oil
- 4 teaspoons sesame seeds
- 2 teaspoons ginger, finely chopped
- A pinch turmeric powder
- Lime juice to taste (optional)
- 2 cups cooked black beans
- 2 cloves garlic, finely minced
- A large pinch red chili flakes
- Salt to taste

Directions:
- Pour enough water to cover the bottom of the saucepan by an inch. Place a strainer on the saucepan. Place broccoli florets on the strainer. Steam the broccoli for 6 minutes.
- Place a large frying pan over medium heat. Add sesame oil. When the oil is just warm, add sesame seeds, chili flakes, ginger, garlic, turmeric powder and salt. Sauté for a couple of minutes until aromatic.
- Add steamed broccoli and black beans and sauté until thoroughly heated.
- Add lime juice and stir.
- Serve hot.

Nutrition:
Calories: 196 kcal
Protein: 11.2 g
Fat: 7.25 g
Carbohydrates: 23.45 g

Hot Pink Coconut Slaw

Preparation Time: 5 minutes
Cooking Time: 0 minutes
Servings: 3
Ingredients:
1. 2 tablespoons lime juice
2. 1 tablespoon olive oil
3. ¼ teaspoon salt
4. 2 cups purple cabbage, thinly sliced
5. ½ small jalapeño, deseeded, discard membranes, chopped
6. ½ cup large coconut flakes, unsweetened or shredded coconut, unsweetened
7. 2 tablespoons apple cider vinegar
8. ½ tablespoon honey or maple syrup
9. 1 cup red onion, thinly sliced
10. ½ cup radish, thinly sliced or shredded carrots
11. ¼ cup fresh cilantro, chopped

Directions:
- Put all together the ingredients into a bowl and toss well. Cover and set aside for 30-40 minutes.
- Toss well and serve.

Nutrition:
Calories: 179 kcal
Protein: 3.92 g
Fat: 10.64 g
Carbohydrates: 18.53 g

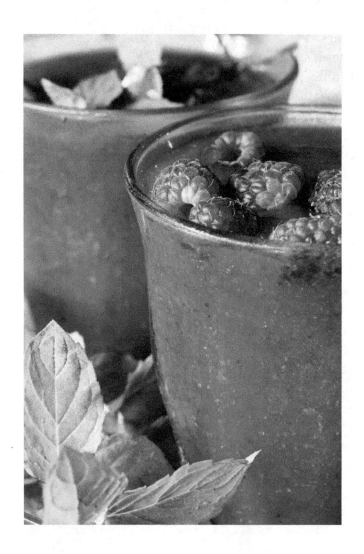

Fresh Strawberry Salsa

Preparation Time: 10 minutes
Cooking Time: 0 minutes
Servings: 6-8
Ingredients:
1. ½ teaspoon lime zest, grated
2. 2 teaspoons pure raw honey
3. 2 kiwi fruit, peeled, chopped
4. ½ cup fresh cilantro
5. ¼ cup fresh lime juice
6. 2 pounds fresh ripe strawberries, hulled, chopped
7. ½ cup red onion, finely chopped
8. 1-2 jalapeños, deseeded, finely chopped

Directions:
- Add lime juice, lime zest and honey into a large bowl and whisk well.
- Add rest of the ingredients then mix well. Cover and set aside for a while for the flavors to set in. Serve.

Nutrition:
Calories: 119 kcal
Protein: 9.26 g
Fat: 4.38 g
Carbohydrates: 11.73 g

Rice with Pistachios

Preparation Time: 10 minutes
Cooking Time: 20 minutes
Servings: 6
Ingredients:
1. 2 dry baby leaves
2. 1 thinly sliced medium onion
3. 5 pods of slightly crushed green cardamom
4. 1 ½ cups of Basmati rice (rinsed in a colander and soaked in water for about 30 minutes, or more)
5. ½ cup of chopped and packed dill leaves
6. ¼ cup of raw pistachios (or more for garnish)
7. 3 cups of vegetable stock or water
8. ½ teaspoon of turmeric
9. 1 teaspoon of vegetable oil
10. Salt, to taste
11. Ground black pepper (to taste)

Directions:
- In a large saucepan, warm the oil and add the cardamom. Heat it for about 1 minute until it turns slightly brown and add the onion. Sauté for about 1-2 minutes.
- Stir in the dill leaves, turmeric and pistachios. Then add the rice and stir-fry for about 1 minute.
- Mix the vegetable stock, black pepper and salt to taste, stir it well and bring it to a boil.
- Cover the pan using lid and cook over medium-low heat for about 15 minutes.
- Take it off from the heat then set aside the rice (covered) for about 10 minutes. Then fluff it with a fork and add more pistachios as garnish, if you desire.
- Enjoy!

Nutrition:
Calories: 90 kcal
Protein: 3.36 g

Fat: 5.08 g
Carbohydrates: 8.39 g

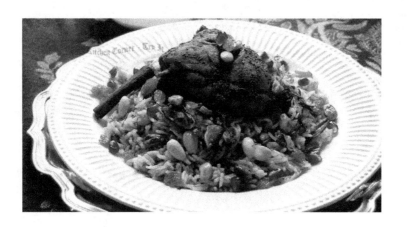

Red Cabbage with Cheese

Preparation Time: 5 minutes
Cooking Time: 12 minutes
Servings: 4
Ingredients:
1. ¼ cup & 1 tbsp. of extra virgin olive oil
2. 8 cups of red cabbage, thinly sliced
3. 1 cup of walnuts
4. 1 Tbsp. of crumbled blue cheese
5. 1 tbsp. of Dijon mustard
6. 3 tbsp. of pure maple syrup
7. 3 tbsp. of red wine vinegar
8. 1 tsp of butter
9. ¼ tsp of salt
10. ¼ tsp of freshly ground pepper
11. 2 thinly sliced scallions

Directions:
- For the vinaigrette:
- Blend the blue cheese, ¼ cup of olive oil, mustard, vinegar, salt, and pepper in a food processor or blender until the mixture has a creamy consistency.
- For the salad:
- Place a parchment paper near the stove.
- Heat 1 tbsp. Of oil over medium heat in a medium-sized skillet and stir in the walnuts, cooking them for about 2 minutes.
- Now mix salt and pepper, drizzle maple syrup and cook for about 3-5 minutes while stirring the mixture up to the nuts are evenly coated.
- Transfer to the paper and pour the remaining syrup over them using a spoon. Separate the nuts and cool down for about 5 minutes.
- In a large bowl, add the cabbage and scallions and toss them with the vinaigrette. Add the walnuts and blue cheese as toppings.

Nutrition:
Calories 232
Fat 19 gram
Saturated Fat 4 gram
Sodium 267 gram
Carbs 12 gram
Fiber 2 gram
Sugar 8 gram
Added sugar 5 gram
Protein 4 gram

Goat Cheese Salad

Preparation Time: 15 minutes
Cooking Time: 30 minutes
Servings:4
Ingredients:
1. 2 tbsp. of red wine vinegar
2. 2 bunches of medium beets (~1 ½ lbs.) with trimmed tops
3. 1 bunch of trimmed and torn arugula
4. Kosher salt + freshly ground black pepper
5. 1/3 cup extra virgin olive oil
6. ½ cup of walnuts
7. ½ head of escarole (medium), torn
8. 4 oz. crumbled of goat cheese (aged cheese is preferred)

Directions:
- Put the beets in water in a saucepan and apply salt as seasoning. Now, boil them over high heat for about 20 minutes or until they're tender. Peel them off when they're cool with your fingers or use a knife.
- To taste, whisk the vinegar with salt and pepper in a large bowl. Then mix in the olive oil for the dressing. Toss the beets with the dressing, so they're evenly coated and marinate them for about 15 minutes – 2 hours.
- Set the oven to 350F. Bring the nuts on a baking sheet and toast them for about 8 minutes (stirring them once) until they turn golden brown. Allow them to cool.
- Mix and toss the escarole and arugula with the beets and place them in four plates. Add the walnuts and goat cheese as toppings and serve.
- Enjoy!

Nutrition:
Calories: 285 kcal
Protein: 11.85 g
Fat: 25.79 g

Carbohydrates: 2.01 g

Cucumber Yogurt Salad with Mint

Preparation Time: 10 minutes
Cooking Time: 0 minutes
Servings: 2
Ingredients:
1. 2 chopped organic cucumbers
2. ½ cup chopped organic red onion
3. ¼ cup organic coconut milk
4. ¼ cup organic mint leaves
5. 1 teaspoon organic dill weed
6. ¼ teaspoon pink Himalayan sea salt
7. 3 tablespoons fresh organic lime juice
8. 1 tablespoon extra virgin olive oil
9. 1 tablespoon plain organic goat yogurt

Directions:
- Chop the red onion, dill, cucumbers, and mint and mix them in a large bowl.
- Blend them until they're smooth.
- Top the dressing onto the cucumber salad and mix thoroughly. Chill for at least 1 hour before you serve.
- Enjoy!

Nutrition:
Calories: 207 kcal
Protein: 6.9 g
Fat: 13.87 g
Carbohydrates: 18.04 g

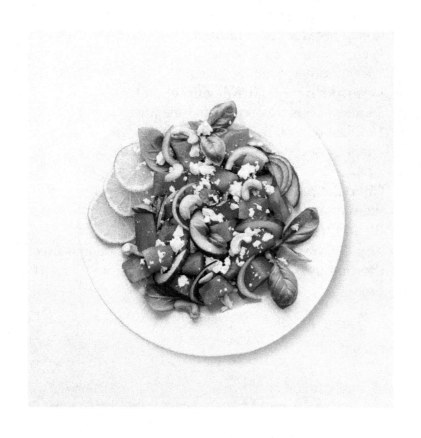

Beet Hummus

Preparation Time: 5 minutes
Cooking Time: 0 minutes
Servings: 2
Ingredients:
1. 1 clove of garlic
2. 1 skinless roasted beet
3. 1 ¾ cup of chickpeas
4. ½ cup of olive oil
5. 2 tbsp. of sunflower seeds
6. Juice of one lemon
7. ¼ tsp of chili flakes
8. 1 ½ tsp of cumin
9. 1 tsp of curry
10. 1 tsp of maple syrup
11. ½ tsp of oregano
12. ½ tsp of salt
13. 1 nub of fresh ginger

Directions:
- Blend all together the ingredients in a food processor until they're smooth and garnish them with sunflower seeds.
- Enjoy!

Nutrition:
Calories: 423 kcal
Protein: 13.98 g
Fat: 24.26 g
Carbohydrates: 40.13 g

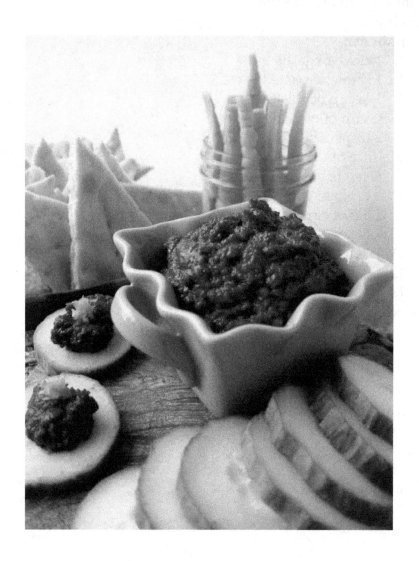

Feta Cheese Salad

Preparation Time: 10 minutes
Cooking Time: 0 minutes
Servings: 2
Ingredients:
1. 4 tomatoes
2. 30 g feta cheese
3. 2 cucumbers
4. 1 tbsp. olive oil (extra virgin)
5. 4 spring onions
6. 1 tsp balsamic vinegar
7. Salt

Directions:
- Cube the tomatoes and cucumbers.
- Thinly slice the onions.
- Crumble the feta cheese.
- Mix tomatoes, onions, and cucumbers.
- Put olive oil, vinegar, and a bit of salt.
- Add feta cheese.
- Enjoy your meal!

Nutrition:
Calories: 221 kcal
Protein: 9.24 g
Fat: 13.84 g
Carbohydrates: 17.18 g

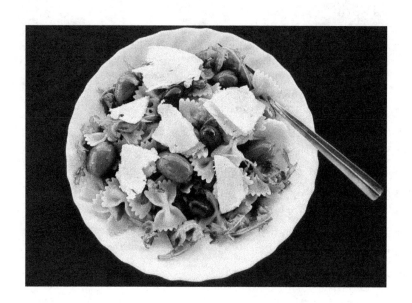

Quinoa Salad

Preparation Time: 10 minutes
Cooking Time: 0 minutes
Servings: 2
Ingredients:
1. ½ cup quinoa (uncooked)
2. 2 brussels sprouts
3. 1 carrot
4. ¼ tsp sea salt
5. 1 tbsp. flaxseed oil
6. 1 tbsp. apple cider vinegar

Directions:
- Rinse quinoa thoroughly.
- Dice the carrots and brussels sprouts to very small pieces.
- Cook the quinoa based on the instruction on the packaging.
- Mix flaxseed oil, sea salt, and apple cider vinegar.
- Sauté brussels sprouts and carrots on a bit of olive oil for a few minutes.
- After both brussels sprouts and carrots, and quinoa are ready, mix them all in a bowl.
- Add the dressing and mix thoroughly.
- Serve warm.

Nutrition:
Calories: 280 kcal
Protein: 10.15 g
Fat: 12.52 g
Carbohydrates: 31.99 g

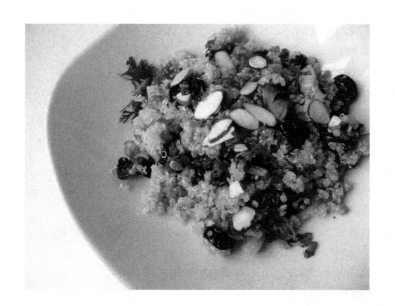

Lentil Salad

Preparation Time: 10 minutes
Cooking Time: 0 minutes
Servings: 2
Ingredients:
1. 2 cups lentil
2. Turmeric – to your taste
3. 1 red bell pepper
4. 3 spring onions
5. 1 tbsp. lime juice
6. ½ cup parsley
7. 1 tbsp. olive oil
8. 15 basil leaves
9. A pinch of salt

Directions:
- Cook the lentils based on the package instructions. Add a garlic clove while cooking.
- When cooled, remove the garlic clove and put the lentils into a large bowl.
- Chop all the vegetables then add them to the lentils.
- Add lime juice, a bit of salt, and olive oil.
- Mix well.

Nutrition:
Calories: 207 kcal
Protein: 11.53 g
Fat: 10.49 g
Carbohydrates: 22.37 g

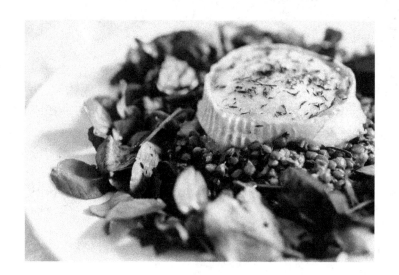

CPSIA information can be obtained
at www.ICGtesting.com
Printed in the USA
BVHW010941210421
605311BV00005B/103

9 781801 757867